To:

From:

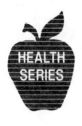

Heart Healthy Favorites
Low Cholesterol Cooking

by Sue E. Willett, Home Economist

Printed in the United States of America
ISBN   1-56383-005-1

Published by G & R Publishing Co.
507 Industrial Street
Waverly, IA 50677

About the Author

Sue Willett graduated with honors from Central State University, Edmond Oklahoma, with a B.S. in Home Economics and a concentration in Business. Since 1985 she has proven her business talents as President of the M.S. Willett Co., Inc.; a leading edge company in product research, design, development and marketing.

In addition to the Health Series, Sue is author or co-author of four books and guides to healthy cooking and eating. After experiencing heart disease in her own family, Sue set about working to help others reduce their risks. Her books bring together lowfat - low cholesterol cooking with today's lifestyles. Ranging from traditional country cuisine to modern microwave dishes these recipes and tips provide for great tasting nutrition.

Sue and her family live in Cedar Falls, Iowa. Her husband and two children have been extremly helpful with taste-testing these recipes.

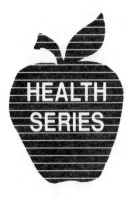

HEALTH SERIES

Fabulous Fiber Favorites
Subtitle: High Fiber Naturally

Kids Eat Healthy
Subtitle: Delicious and Nutritious

On A Healthy Wok
Subtitle: Quick and Easy

Microwave Cooking
Subtitle: Low Cholesterol and Lowfat

Healthy Entertaining
Subtitle: Here's To Your Health!

Heart Healthy Favorites
Subtitle: Low Cholesterol Cooking

Sweet & Natural
"Fruit Sweetened"

Unibook Series

1100	Cookies	2200	Beef	3700	Cajun
1200	Casseroles	2300	Holiday Collection	3800	Household Hints
1300	Meat Dishes	2400	Salads & Dressings	6100	Chinese
1400	Microwave	2500	Wild Game	6400	German
1500	Cooking for "2"	2600	Soups	6700	Italian
1600	Slow Cooking	3100	Fish & Seafood	6800	Irish
1700	Low Calorie	3200	Poultry	7000	Mexican
1900	Pastries & Pies	3300	My Own Recipes	7100	Norwegian
2000	Outdoor Grilling	3400	Low Cholesterol	7200	Swedish
2100	Appetizers	3500	Chocoholic		

TABLE OF CONTENTS

HEART HEALTHY COOKING

Heart disease is the <u>Number One</u> killer in this country today. However, unlike many other causes of death, heart disease may be largely avoidable. We can reduce our risk of heart disease dramatically just by making more healthful food choices. As individuals, we can play a very active role in our own health maintenance by: maintaining our ideal body weight; decreasing our consumption of fat, cholesterol and salt; not smoking; getting regular exercise; and keeping an eye on our blood cholesterol levels. Research has proven that high levels of blood cholesterol increase our risk of heart disease!

WHAT IS CHOLESTEROL?

Cholesterol is a complex fat-like substance. We get it in two ways, directly from the foods we eat, and from within our own bodies. Cholesterol is produced naturally in the liver. All animals produce cholesterol, thus any food that is an

I

animal product will contain a certain amount of it. The body uses cholesterol for a number of functions, however too much in the system can be harmful. The primary problem occurs when there is excess cholesterol in the blood. That which is not used is deposited on the artery walls. As it builds up, blood flow can be restricted or even blocked altogether. Thus keeping blood cholesterol levels low is vital to maintaining a healthy circulatory system.

Choosing the right kinds of foods is an important first step in getting cholesterol under control. Do your heart a favor - Start making healthy food choices today!

Since dietary fat is an important factor in determining cholesterol level, here is some information on the types of fat:

SATURATED FATS: These are fats that are solid at room temperature. They can be found in animal products, and tropical plant oils. Saturated fats tend to raise blood cholesterol levels.

UNSATURATED FATS: These include both polyunsaturated and monounsaturated oils. They come from plants and plant products. Both types may actually help to reduce blood cholesterol levels.

POLYUNSATURATED FATS are oils from certain vegetable products. They are usually liquid at room temperature. Examples are sunflower, safflower, corn and soybean oil.

MONOUNSATURATED FATS are also vegetable oils that are liquid at room temperature. Examples are canola and olive oil.

HEART HEALTHY GUIDELINES FOR FAT CONSUMPTION

1. Fat should account for only about 30% of total calorie intake:
   10% saturated fats,
   10% polyunsaturated fats,
   10% monounsaturated fats.

2. Cholesterol should be limited to 300 milligrams per day.
3. Reduce sodium intake. The body's sodium requirements are generally met without any added salt in the diet.

TIPS FOR LIMITING FAT INTAKE

1. Cut back on fried foods.

2. Cut back on high fat snacks such as chips, doughnuts, cakes, pies and cookies.

3. Eat more fruits, vegetables, whole grains, and lowfat dairy products and meats.

4. Use less dressing, sauce or gravy.

5. Reduce portion sizes, and don't always go back for seconds.

6. Substitute two egg whites for one whole egg in recipes.

7. Trim the visible fat from meats, cut the skin from poultry.

8. Use plain lowfat yogurt in place of sour cream.

9. Broil, roast or bake meats instead of pan frying.

10. Read the labels! When shopping, look for products that are lower in fat, cholesterol and sodium.

LOW CHOLESTEROL FOODS:

Egg whites	"GOOD OILS":
Fish	Canola oil
Frozen lowfat yogurt	Corn oil
Fruits Cottonseed oil	Olive oil

V

Lean meats
Low meat main dishes
Lowfat cottage cheese
Lowfat crackers and snacks
Lowfat whole grain breads
Lowfat yogurt
Pasta made without eggs
Pumpkin seeds
Sesame seeds
Sherbet
Skim milk
Sunflower seeds
Vegetables
Wild game

Safflower oil
Sesame oil
Sunflower oil

MARGARINES:
Soft, tub, squeeze or diet
Check the label!

TIPS FOR EATING IN A RESTAURANT

1. Look for lowfat and fat-free foods. Examples include vegetables, fruits, legumes and grains.

2. Ask how the food is prepared. Choose broiled or poached items over fried or batter dipped. The more simply prepared the item, the better!

3. Look for descriptions such as: steamed, poached, roasted, fresh from the garden, in its own juice, in a tomato sauce, or broiled in lemon juice; and choose items that are prepared in these ways.

4. Avoid foods that are: creamed, in gravy, sauteed, fried, buttered, in butter sauce, escalloped, casseroled, au gratin, or marinated in oil or cheese sauce.

5. Drink skim milk instead of whole milk, or a shake.

6. Watch for saturated fats. Avoid fatty meats, lard and butter. Select instead small amounts of polyunsaturated fats such as margarine for your dinner roll.

7. Always ask for dressings and sauces on the side, and use less of them.

8. If the restaurant hasn't already done so, trim the fat from meats, remove the skin from poultry.

9. Choose smaller portions of meat entrees.

10. Select fresh fruits for dessert.

11. Avoid non-dairy creamers and whipped toppings.

12. Try raw vegetables and fresh fruits as appetizers.

13. Salads containing fresh greens, vegetables and fruits are great choices. Lemon juice makes a tasty fat-free dressing.

14. Skip the sour cream on your baked potato, or try lowfat yogurt instead.

15. Select vegetable side dishes that are steamed rather than prepared in butter.

16. At the salad bar go easy on the cheese, pasta salads, potato salads, coleslaw and creamy fruit mixtures.

17. Try honey on rolls instead of butter or margarine.

18. Choose sandwiches without cheese.

19. Skip the french fries at the fast food restaurant - have a salad instead?

SUBSTITUTION CHART

INGREDIENT:	SUBSTITUTION:
EGGS	Use 2 teaspoons polyunsaturated oil and 1 egg white. There are also cholesterol-free egg substitutes on the market.
WHOLE MILK	Skim Milk or non-fat dry milk.
BUTTER	Polyunsaturated margarine or oil.
SOUR CREAM	Lowfat yogurt. Try blended lowfat cottage cheese. Also try mixing ½ cup lowfat cottage cheese, ½ tablespoon lemon juice and 1 tablespoon skim milk.

X

WHIPPED CREAM

Use ¼ cup non-fat dry milk with 1½ tablespoons sugar, 1½ tablespoons oil, ½ teaspoon gelatin, 1 teaspoon cold water, 1½ tablespoons boiling water and ¼ cup ice water.

First mix gelatin with cold water. Stir and add boiling water until it dissolves. Beat non-fat dry milk and ice water in cold bowl on high until it peaks. Still beating add sugar, oil and gelatin. Place in refrigerator until ready.

CREAM CHEESE

Blend ½ cup dry lowfat cottage cheese and 2 tablespoons margarine. You may add a small amount of skim milk in blending.

BUTTERMILK	Beat together briskly 2 cups lukewarm skim milk and 2 tablespoons lemon juice.
HOLLANDAISE SAUCE	Slowly beat 4 tablespoons hot water with 1 cup low calorie mayonnaise. Stir until heated through. Add 2 tablespoons lemon juice. Pour over favorite vegetables.
SALT	Combine 1 tablespoon paprika, 1 tablespoon garlic powder, 1 tablespoon onion powder, 1 tablespoon dry mustard, ½ tablespoon white pepper, 1 teaspoon crushed basil, and ½ teaspoon ground thyme.

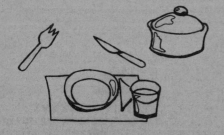

BREADS

APPLESAUCE AND SPICE BREAD

2 C. all-purpose flour
1 tsp. baking soda
½ tsp. baking powder
½ tsp. cinnamon
¼ tsp. salt
¼ tsp. nutmeg
¼ tsp. allspice
1 C. sugar
½ C. vegetable oil

1¼ C. sweetened
  applesauce
½ C. egg substitute
3 T. milk
½ C. coarsely chopped
  walnuts
TOPPING:
¼ C. chopped walnuts
¼ C. packed brown sugar
½ tsp. cinnamon

Sift flour with baking soda, baking powder, salt and spices. Combine sugar, oil, applesauce, egg substitute and milk. Add sifted dry ingredients and nuts. Pour batter into greased 9x5x3" loaf pan. Mix topping ingredients thoroughly and sprinkle over batter. Bake at 350° for 1¼ hours. Makes 1 loaf.

BANANA BREAD

1½ C. all-purpose flour
1 tsp. baking soda
1 C. sugar
¼ tsp. salt
4 bananas, mashed

½ C. egg substitute
1 tsp. vanilla
½ C. safflower oil
¾ C. plain nonfat yogurt
⅔ C. raisins
Margarine

Sift together flour, soda, sugar and salt; set aside. Blend bananas, egg substitute, vanilla and oil in blender; add yogurt and raisins. Pour over dry ingredients. Blend with wire whisk until smooth. Pour into a loaf pan greased with margarine. Bake at 350° for 1 hour.

BANANA MUFFINS

2¼ C. oat-bran cereal
1 T. baking powder
¼ C. brown sugar
¼ C. chopped pecans

1¼ C. skim milk
2 ripe bananas
2 egg whites
2 T. vegetable oil

Blend dry ingredients in a large bowl. Mix the milk, bananas, egg whites and oil in a bowl or blender. Add to the dry ingredients and mix. Line the muffin pan with paper baking cups and fill them with batter. Bake for 17 minutes at 425°.

BANANA NUT BREAD

½ C. softened margarine
1 C. well-packed brown sugar
2 egg whites
3 T. skim milk, orange or
   apple juice
1 C. ripe mashed bananas

2½ tsp. baking powder
¼ tsp. salt
2 C. whole wheat flour
½ C. nuts
1 tsp. vanilla
¼ tsp. almond flavoring

Cream margarine and brown sugar. Add vanilla and almond flavorings; beat in egg whites. Stir together flour; baking powder and salt. Add liquid and bananas to creamed mixture. Stir in flour, add nuts and pour in two greased and floured loaf pans (approximately 8x4x2½"). Bake at 350° for 50 to 60 minutes or until bread pulls away from pan.

BLUEBERRY COFFEE CAKE

¾ C. sugar
¼ C. margarine
¼ C. egg substitute or
  2 egg whites
¾ C. milk
1 tsp. vanilla

½ tsp. salt
3 tsp. baking powder
1½ C. drained blueberries
4 T. sugar
½ tsp. cinnamon
2 C. flour

Cream sugar and margarine. Add vanilla and egg substitute. Blend flour, salt and baking powder; add alternately with milk. Mix only long enough to blend. Spread half the batter in 9x9" pan. Cover with blueberries and 2 tablespoons sugar. Spread rest of batter and top with 2 tablespoons sugar and cinnamon. Bake at 350° for 35 to 40 minutes.

BLUEBERRY BREAKFAST BREAD

¼ C. margarine
½ C. sugar
1 egg, slightly beaten or
  2 egg whites
1 carton plain or vanilla
  lowfat yogurt
½ tsp. vanilla
2 C. flour, (½ to 1 C. of whole
  wheat, if desired)

2 tsp. baking powder
½ pt. blueberries,
  rinsed, dried
  and lightly dusted with flour
STREUSEL TOPPING:
¼ C. flour
¼ C. sugar
1 tsp. cinnamon
2 T. margarine

Preheat oven to 350°. Cream ¼ cup margarine and ½ cup sugar. Add egg, yogurt and vanilla. Sift together flour(s) and baking powder. Add dry ingredients to creamed mixture just until moistened and fold in blueberries. Pour batter into 5x9" well-greased loaf pan. Combine ingredients for topping until crumbly. Sprinkle over top and lightly swirl through with a knife. Bake for 1 hour until toothpick inserted comes out clean and is lightly browned. Can be frozen.

CINNAMON APPLE COFFEE CAKE

¼ C. egg substitute or
  2 egg whites
⅓ C. sugar
1 C. sifted flour
3 tsp. baking powder
½ tsp. salt
½ C. skim milk
1 C. rolled oats
¼ C. melted margarine

2 (or more) lg. cooking
  apples, sliced
Pecan halves or other nuts
TOPPING:
½ tsp. cinnamon
¼ C. sugar
¼ tsp. nutmeg
2 T. melted margarine

Beat egg substitute or 2 egg whites and sugar until light and fluffy. Add flour, baking powder, salt and milk; stir lightly. Add in oatmeal and melted margarine. Spread half of batter in a greased 9" round pan. Cover batter with a layer of thinly sliced apples. Spread the remaining batter on top. (The apples will show through.) Mix topping dry ingredients and sprinkle over top of cake. Pour the melted margarine over the top of this. Decorate with the nuts. Bake at 350° for 30 to 40 minutes. Serve warm.

BLUEBERRY RAISIN BRAN MUFFINS

1 stick margarine
1 C. sugar
½ C. egg substitute
2½ C. flour
2½ tsp. baking soda
2 C. buttermilk (see
   substitution chart)

1 C. 100% Bran
1 C. boiling water
2 C. All Bran
½ C. chopped nuts
½ C. raisins
½ C. blueberries

Cream margarine with sugar and egg substitute. Sift flour with baking soda and add to first mixture, alternating with buttermilk substitute; mix well. Combine 100% Bran and boiling water. Let stand for 1 minute. Add this to mixture and stir thoroughly. Then fold in All Bran, nuts, raisins and blueberries. Make 24 muffins. Bake at 400° for 15 minutes.

EGG SUBSTITUTE KOLACHES

2 yeast cakes or 2 pkgs.
  dry yeast
1 C. warm water
½ C. sugar
1 C. corn oil margarine

½ tsp. salt
1 C. cold water
¾ C. egg substitute or
  equivalent to 3 eggs
6½ C. flour

Dissolve yeast in the warm water in small bowl. Melt margarine in large glass bowl in microwave, add sugar and salt; stir until sugar is dissolved. Add the cold water, dissolved yeast and egg substitutes to margarine mixture and mix with egg beater. Stir in flour and allow to double in refrigerator overnight or 6 hours. Grease cookie sheet with corn oil margarine and place walnut sized dough balls on sheet 1½" apart. Brush with melted margarine. Let rise until light. Punch down center of dough with fingers and fill with your favorite filling. Bake at 400° for 8 to 10 minutes. This dough can be used for tea rings and rolls.

FRUIT MUFFINS

2¼ C. oat-bran cereal
1 T. baking powder
¼ C. raisins
2 T. vegetable oil
1 C. evaporated skim milk

2 egg whites
1-16 oz. can pears, peaches
  or fruit cocktail, drained

Blend dry ingredients in a bowl. Mix together other ingredients, except the
fruit. Add the liquid mixture to the dry ingredients and mix. Chop the canned
fruit fine and add to the batter. If the batter seems dry, add a bit of the fluid
drained from the fruit. Line the muffin pan with paper baking cups and fill
with batter. Bake at 425° for 17 minutes.

OLD-FASHIONED PANCAKES

1 C. egg substitute
1 C. skim milk
1 C. cold water
2½ C. flour, sifted

¼ C. safflower oil
¾ tsp. sugar
¼ tsp. salt
Blueberries, optional

Beat egg substitute, milk and water lightly; add remaining ingredients. Mix with a wire whisk. Bake on a preheated griddle. Turn pancakes when top side is bubbly. To make blueberry pancakes, just after bubbles have broken, sprinkle pancakes with blueberries. Turn and brown on other side.

13

PARKER HOUSE DINNER ROLLS

¾ C. skim milk
2 T. sugar
1¼ tsp. salt
1 pkg. yeast

¾ C. lukewarm water
¼ C. oil
4 C. sifted flour

After bringing milk to boil, add sugar and salt. Cool to lukewarm. Add the yeast to the water for 5 minutes; stir in the milk mixture and the oil. Beat in 2 cups flour until smooth. Add enough of the remaining flour to make a soft dough. Knead on a lightly floured surface until smooth. Place in a lightly oiled bowl, brush top with oil, cover and set in a warm place to rise until double in bulk. Punch dough down on a lightly floured surface and divide in half. Roll each half into a circle ½" thick. Cut into 2" rounds. Crease dough heavily with the dull edge of a knife through the center and brush lightly with oil. Fold over into pocketbook shape. Arrange on an oiled baking sheet, leaving 1" between each. Cover and let rise in a warm place for 1 hour. Bake at 400° for 12 minutes or until browned. Makes 2 dozen.
14

PEACH MUFFINS

½ C. peaches, chopped
⅓ C. margarine
½ C. sugar
1 egg or 2 egg whites
1½ C. flour
1½ tsp. baking powder
½ tsp. salt

¼ tsp. nutmeg
½ C. skim milk
TOPPING:
½ C. sugar
1 tsp. cinnamon
½ C. melted margarine

Cream margarine and sugar. Add egg and mix. Stir in flour, baking powder, salt and nutmeg alternately with milk. Stir in peaches. Fill greased muffin cups ⅔ full. Bake at 350° for 20 to 25 minutes.

TOPPING: Mix cinnamon and sugar. As soon as muffins are done, dip the tops in melted margarine and then in cinnamon-sugar mixture. Serve warm. Makes 12 muffins.

WHITE BREAD

1 pkg. yeast	2 T. sugar
¼ C. lukewarm water	¾ tsp. salt
2 C. scalded and cooled	1 T. oil
skim milk	6½ C. sifted flour

Place yeast in the water for 5 minutes. Blend milk, sugar, salt and oil; add 2 cups flour. Mix until smooth. Work in the yeast, then add enough of the remaining flour to make a firm dough. Knead on a lightly floured surface until smooth. Place in a lightly oiled bowl and brush the top with a little oil. Cover and let rise in a warm place until double in bulk. Punch down, cover and let rise again for 45 minutes. Divide dough in 2 pieces, shape each into a ball. Let stand for 10 minutes. Shape into 2 loaves and place in 2 oiled 10" loaf pans. Let rise until double in bulk. Bake at 400° for 50 minutes or until browned and slightly pulling away from the sides of the pan. Cool on rack.

WHOLE WHEAT BREAD

½ C. corn oil margarine
½ C. honey
3 C. stone ground whole
  wheat flour

2 pkgs. dry yeast, dissolved
  in 2½ C. warm water
1 tsp. salt
5 C. flour, enriched

Mix all ingredients. Let raise for 1 hour. Divide into 3 parts for 3 loaves. Let raise in bread pans until doubled. Bake at 375° for 30 minutes.

ZUCCHINI MUFFINS

3 C. flour
1 tsp. baking powder
1 tsp. baking soda
½ tsp. salt
1 tsp. ground cinnamon
1 C. egg substitute

2 C. sugar
1 C. oil
2 C. grated zucchini
½ tsp. vanilla
1 C. pecans, chopped
½ C. raisins

Combine flour, baking powder, soda, salt and cinnamon in bowl. Beat egg substitute with sugar in large bowl at medium speed for 2 minutes. Gradually add oil, beating constantly for 2 to 3 minutes. Add zucchini and vanilla; blend well. Stir in nuts and raisins. Fold in flour mixture just until batter is evenly moistened. Spoon batter into sprayed muffin pans ⅔ full. Bake in preheated oven at 375° for 25 minutes or until lightly browned. Let stand for 10 minutes. Turn out on racks to cool.

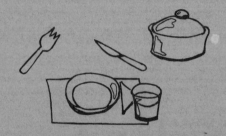

MAIN DISHES

BAKED BREAST OF CHICKEN

3 whole chicken breasts
3 T. flour
½ tsp. salt
½ tsp. freshly ground black
  pepper
3 T. special oil
1 clove garlic, minced

1 C. frozen peas, thawed
½ lb. mushrooms, chopped
2 T. minced parsley
½ C. sliced celery
1 bay leaf
6 lg. lettuce leaves

Halve chicken breasts and remove fat. Rub with flour, salt and pepper mixture. Heat the oil in a deep skillet. Brown the chicken in it. Mix in the garlic; spread the peas, mushrooms, parsley and celery over the chicken. Place the bay leaf in the pan and cover all with the lettuce leaves. Bake in a 350° oven 35 minutes or until tender.

BAKED CHICKEN WITH OIL AND LEMON

2 chicken breasts, halved
2 T. safflower oil
2 T. olive oil
¼ C. fresh lemon juice

1 clove garlic, minced
¼ tsp. oregano
¼ tsp. tarragon

Debone and skin breasts. Mix safflower oil, olive oil, lemon juice, garlic, oregano and tarragon; pour over chicken. Marinate 20 minutes. Bake at 350° for 35 to 45 minutes or until done. Baste frequently during baking.

BAKED TUNA CAKES

4 oz. tuna, drained
¼ tsp. dehydrated onion flakes
¼ C. tomato juice
2 T. chopped celery

Salt and pepper, to taste
1 T. Worcestershire sauce,
  low sodium
1 tsp. prepared mustard

Combine all ingredients and form into 2 patties. Bake at 350° in a non-stick pan, about 30 minutes.

BELIEVE IT OR NOT QUICHE

1 C. egg substitute
½ C. biscuit mix
⅓ C. melted margarine
1½ C. skim milk
Pepper to taste

1 T. dehydrated onion flakes
4 oz. shredded lowfat,
  low sodium yellow cheese
½ C. lean chopped ham

Place all ingredients, except cheese and ham in blender. Mix for a few seconds to blend well. Pour into 9" pie pan that has been greased with non-stick spray. Sprinkle cheese and meat over top and push gently below surface with back of spoon.

For Conventional Oven: Bake at 350° for 45 minutes. Allow to set for 10 minutes before cutting.

For Microwave: Use 50% (medium) power; microwave 15 to 20 minutes until knife inserted comes out clean and quiche seems set, rotating ¼ turn after each ¼ cooking time. Let stand for 10 minutes before cutting. Yield: 8 servings.

BROILED CHICKEN

4-1 lb. broiler halves
½ C. vegetable oil
½ tsp. garlic powder
½ tsp. ground thyme

½ tsp. ground oregano
¾ tsp. salt
⅛ tsp. white pepper

Prepare chicken by washing and trim fat. Mix remaining ingredients and mix well. Brush the broiler halves with the seasoned oil. Place them on a foil-lined broiler rack. Broil 6" to 8" from heat, turning and brushing with seasoned oil as necessary, until the chicken is brown and tender. This will take about 25 to 30 minutes depending upon the amount of heat.

BUTTERMILK MARINATED CHICKEN

2-2½ lb. fryers, disjointed
1 C. buttermilk
1 tsp. salt
¼ tsp. freshly ground black
 pepper

2 cloves, minced
2 T. special oil
1 C. chopped onions
2 T. curry powder
2 T. ground blanched almonds

Wash and dry the chickens; remove any visible fat. Marinate 2 hours in a mixture of the buttermilk, salt, pepper and garlic, turning and basting frequently. Drain chicken well; reserve the marinade. Heat the oil in a deep skillet or casserole; saute the onions 10 minutes. Mix in the curry powder; add the chicken and brown lightly. Add the marinade; cover and cook over low heat 1 hour or until tender. Stir in the almonds; cook 2 minutes. Serves 8.

CAJUN FISH BAKE

⅓ C. low calorie salad dressing
½ tsp. ground cumin
½ tsp. onion powder
¼ tsp. ground red pepper
¼ tsp. garlic powder
1 lb. fish fillets
½ C. crushed sesame
  crackers

Baking Time: 30 minutes for conventional oven or 7 to 8 minutes for microwave oven.

Mix salad dressing and seasonings. Brush fish with salad dressing mixture; coat with crumbs. Place in greased 13x9" baking dish. Bake at 350° for 30 minutes or until fish flakes easily with fork. Makes 3 to 4 servings.

To Microwave: Coat fish with salad dressing mixture as directed. Arrange fish in shallow baking dish, placing thickest portions towards outside of dish. Cover with plastic wrap; vent. Microwave on high for 5 minutes, turning dish after 3 minutes. Let stand, covered for 2 to 3 minutes or until fish flakes easily with fork.

CAJUN PORK ROAST

2 lb. boneless single loin pork
   roast, very lean
Cooking oil
CAJUN SEASONING:
3 T. paprika
½ tsp. red pepper (cayenne)
1 T. garlic powder

2 tsp. oregano
2 tsp. thyme
Pinch of salt
½ tsp. white pepper, ground
½ tsp. cumin
¼ tsp. nutmeg

Rub surface of loin lightly with oil. Combine seasoning mixture and rub well over all surfaces of roast. Place roast in shallow pan and roast in 350° oven for about 1 hour, until internal temperature is 155°. Remove from oven and let rest for 5 to 10 minutes before slicing. Serves 4 to 6.

CAULIFLOWER AND HAM

1 sm. cauliflower, separated into
small bits
3 T. Minute tapioca
½ tsp. salt or less
⅛ tsp. pepper
⅛ tsp paprika

2 C. skim milk
2 T. margarine
½ lb. ham (96% fat free),
cubed
½ C. margarined bread
crumbs, finely crumbled

Cook cauliflower in boiling water for 5 minutes; drain. Combine tapioca, salt, pepper, paprika and milk in top of double boiler. Place over rapidly boiling water. Cook for 8 to 10 minutes; add margarine. Place layer of tapioca mix in greased baking dish. Add layer of cauliflower, top with ham, repeat layers with tapioca on top. Cover with crumbs. Bake at 350° for 20 minutes.

CHICKEN ALA KING

2 T. special oil
¾ C. diced green peppers
½ lb. mushrooms
3 C. cubed, cooked chicken
3 pimentos

2 T. cornstarch
3 C. chicken broth
1 egg yolk
2 T. dry sherry

Saute the green peppers 5 minutes in oil. Add the mushrooms; saute 5 minutes. Mix in the chicken and pimentos. Keep warm while preparing the sauce. Mix the cornstarch with the broth until smooth. Cook over low heat, stirring steadily to the boiling point. Cook 5 minutes longer. Beat the egg yolk and sherry in a bowl; slowly add the hot sauce, stirring steadily to prevent curdling. Return to the saucepan; mix in the chicken mixture. Heat but do not boil. Serve over toast or rice.

CHICKEN AND NOODLES

2 whole raw chicken breasts
4 T. special oil
¾ C. thinly sliced onions
2 C. sliced celery
2 C. bean sprouts
½ tsp. salt
¼ tsp. freshly ground black
  pepper

2 T. low salt soy sauce
½ tsp. sugar
1 T. cornstarch
¾ C. chicken broth
1½ C. cooked, drained fine
  noodles (see homemade
  noodle recipe)

Debone and skin chicken; cut into narrow strips. Heat the oil in a deep skillet; saute the chicken 5 minutes. Mix in the onions, celery, bean sprouts, salt, pepper, soy sauce and sugar. Cover and cook over low heat for 8 minutes. Blend the cornstarch and broth; stir into the skillet until thickened. Add the noodles and stir. Cook 2 minutes only.

CHICKEN CACCIATORE

3½ lb. fryer, cut-up
3 T. flour
¾ tsp. salt
½ tsp. freshly ground black
  pepper
2 T. special oil
¾ C. chopped onions

2 C. canned Italian-style
  tomatoes
1 green pepper, diced
½ C. sliced mushrooms
¼ tsp. oregano
¼ C. dry red wine
2 T. minced parsley

Trim visible fat from chicken. Toss with the flour, salt and pepper. Heat the oil in a deep skillet or casserole; brown the chicken and onions in it. Add the tomatoes, green pepper, mushrooms, oregano and wine. Cover and cook over low heat 50 minutes or until tender. Sprinkle with the parsley.

CHICKEN CACCIATORE WITH MACARONI

1-28 oz. can tomatoes
1 T. oil
1 onion, chopped
3 carrots, peeled and thinly
   sliced
3 stalks celery, thinly sliced
2 T. red wine vinegar

¼ tsp. pepper
¾ tsp. sage
¼ tsp. salt
¼ tsp. sugar
2 chicken breasts, halved
¾ lb. shell-shaped macaroni

Mix all ingredients, except chicken and pasta in a pot; bring to a boil. Reduce heat; cover and simmer 25 to 30 minutes. Skin and debone chicken; add to sauce and cook 25 to 30 minutes or until tender. Serve over cooked pasta.

CHICKEN CASSEROLE

2-1¼ lbs. broilers, quartered	1 bay leaf
¾ tsp. salt	½ tsp. thyme
¼ tsp. white pepper	1 T. cornstarch
2 T. special oil	1 C. chicken broth
2 cloves	1 pkg. frozen peas, thawed
8 sm. white onions	½ tsp. sugar
6 peppercorns	⅛ tsp. nutmeg

Remove fat from chicken. Season with salt and pepper. Heat the oil in a casserole. Place the chicken in it. Stick the cloves in an onion and add with all the onions, the peppercorns, bay leaf and thyme. Cover and bake in a 350° oven for 30 minutes. Skim the fat. Mix the cornstarch with the broth; add to the casserole with the peas, sugar and nutmeg. Recover and bake 35 minutes longer or until chicken is tender.

CHICKEN CHOW MEIN

2 T. special oil
1½ C. thinly sliced onions
2 C. sliced celery
¾ lb. mushrooms
1½ C. chicken broth

1 C. bean sprouts
1 C. sliced water chestnuts
1 T. cornstarch
3 T. low salt soy sauce
2 C. cooked chicken

Saute onions in oil for 5 minutes. Add the celery and mushrooms; saute 5 minutes. Blend in the broth, bean sprouts and water chestnuts; cook 3 minutes. Blend cornstarch and soy sauce together. Stir into the vegetable mixture until thickened. Add the chicken. Heat and serve with fine, boiled noodles. (See homemade noodle recipe.)

CHICKEN HASH

2 T. special margarine
½ C. chopped onion
1½ C. peeled, diced potatoes
2 C. diced, cooked chicken

½ tsp. salt
¼ tsp. freshly ground black
 pepper
½ C. chicken broth
1 T. minced parsley

Saute onions and potatoes 10 minutes in melted margarine. Add the chicken, salt and pepper; cook 1 minute. Blend in the broth and parsley; cook over low heat 10 minutes. Serves 6.

CHICKEN ON A STICK

1-8 oz. container plain
  lowfat yogurt
½ C. finely chopped onion
1 clove garlic, minced
1½ tsp. paprika
¾ tsp. ground coriander
¼ tsp. salt

8 boneless chicken breast
  halves, skinned or 12
  chicken thighs,
  skinned and boned
2 lg. red sweet peppers,
  seeded and cut into
  1¼" squares

In medium bowl, mix together first 6 ingredients. Spread half of the mixture in bottom of 8x12" baking dish. Cut each boneless breast half crosswise into thirds; or cut each boned thigh in half. Place chicken pieces in single layer on top of yogurt mixture in baking dish. Spread with remaining yogurt mixture. Cover and marinate in refrigerator overnight. Thread chicken pieces and red pepper squares onto 8 skewers. Grill over medium-hot coals, turning occasionally, until chicken is no longer pink in center and juices run clear, about 18 minutes. Makes 8 servings.   35

CHICKEN PILAF

1½ C. raw rice
1-3½ lb. fryer, cut-up
4 T. special oil
1 C. thinly sliced onions
1½ C. buttermilk, lowfat

½ tsp. salt
¼ tsp. white pepper
½ tsp. powdered ginger
2 C. hot chicken broth
1 green pepper

Cover rice with water and bring to a boil; let stand 15 minutes, then drain well. Wash and dry the chicken; remove fat. Heat the oil in a casserole and brown the chicken and onions in it. Add the buttermilk, salt, pepper and ginger; bring to a boil and cook over low heat 20 minutes. Add the rice and broth and arrange the green peppers on top. Cover and cook over low heat 35 minutes.

CHICKEN-POTATO PIE

3 C. diced, cooked chicken
1 C. cooked peas
2 egg whites, beaten
½ C. chicken broth
2 T. dry bread crumbs
2 T. minced parsley

2 C. mashed potatoes
2 T. special margarine, melted
½ C. hot skim milk
¾ tsp. salt
¼ tsp. white pepper
⅛ tsp. nutmeg

Blend chicken, peas, egg, broth, bread crumbs and parsley. Put into a deep 9" pie plate. Beat until light and fluffy the potatoes, margarine, milk, salt, pepper and nutmeg. Spread over the chicken, covering the edges. Bake in a 375° oven 30 minutes or until browned. Serves 6.

CHICKEN SCAMPI

2 tsp. margarine
⅛ C. olive oil
¼ C. chopped onions
1 T. minced garlic
Juice of 1 lemon
2 lb. chicken breasts,
  skinned and cut into ½"
  pieces

½ tsp. salt
½ tsp. pepper
¼ C. fresh parsley
3 tomatoes, chopped
Hot noodles or rice

In skillet, heat oil and margarine together. Saute onion and garlic briefly. Add lemon juice, chicken, salt, pepper and parsley. Cook, stirring frequently, with lid on until chicken is white and well cooked. Add tomatoes and heat through. Serve over noodles or rice. Makes 4 to 6 servings.

CHICKEN WITH MUSHROOM SAUCE

2 whole med. chicken breasts,
  1½ lbs., skinned, boned and
  halved lengthwise
½ C. evaporated skim milk
1 C. fine dry whole wheat
  bread crumbs
2 C. sliced fresh mushrooms

2 T. sliced green onion
½ C. dry white wine
1 tsp. lemon juice
⅛ tsp. dried thyme, crushed
⅛ tsp. dried marjoram, crushed

Flatten chicken breasts. Dip in milk, then in bread crumbs. Roll up jelly roll style. Place in an 8x8x2" baking pan. Bake, covered, in a 350° oven for 20 minutes. Meanwhile, for sauce, in a skillet combine mushrooms, onion, wine, lemon juice, thyme and marjoram. Cook until vegetables are tender. Spoon sauce into dish with chicken. Bake, uncovered, for 5 minutes more or until chicken is done. To serve, spoon sauce over chicken. Makes 4 servings.

CHICKEN WITH RICE AND PEAS

3 lbs. chicken breasts and
   thighs
3 T. vegetable oil
2 C. chopped canned
   tomatoes and juice
1 C. hot water
2 chicken bouillon cubes
1 C. sliced onions

2 T. chopped parsley
1 tsp. salt
¼ tsp. pepper
½ tsp. basil leaves
½ tsp. garlic powder
1½ C. long grain rice
1-10 oz. pkg. frozen peas

Wash the chicken, drain it and remove its fat and skin with a sharp knife. Saute the chicken in oil in heavy saucepan until lightly browned. Add the tomatoes, water, bouillon cubes, onions, parsley, salt, pepper, basil and garlic powder. Cover and simmer it over a low heat for 20 minutes. Add the rice and simmer for 15 minutes, add the peas and simmer another 10 minutes, or until done and liquid is absorbed. (Add extra water at the end of the cooking if necessary.) Serve hot in shallow soup bowls. Serves 6.   40

CRISPY OVEN-FRIED CHICKEN

2 chicken breast, cut in half   *½ C. Grape-Nuts Flakes*
½ C. skim milk

Trim skin from chicken. Dip chicken in milk, then in Grape-Nuts Flakes. Bake in a Teflon pan at 400° for ½ hour. Reduce heat to 350°. Cover loosely with foil. Bake 20 to 30 minutes longer. Do not turn chicken during baking.

CURRIED CHICKEN AND PASTA

1 lb. (2 C.) skinless, cooked, cubed chicken
2 C. cooked pasta
¼ C. diced fresh red peppers
¼ C. chopped walnuts
½ C. plain lowfat or non-fat yogurt
Salt and pepper, if desired

¼ C. mock sour cream
2 T. curry powder
½ tsp. cumin
1 clove minced garlic
¼ tsp. red pepper sauce
1 T. chopped parsley

In medium bowl, combine chicken, pasta, red peppers and walnuts. For dressing, combine yogurt, mock sour cream, curry, cumin, garlic and red pepper sauce in small bowl. Stir dressing into chicken mixture. Salt and pepper, to taste. Garnish with chopped parsley.

VARIATION: Add ¼ cup cooked, chilled peas or ¼ cup raisins.

EASY OVEN-FRIED CHICKEN

1 chicken breast per person
Safflower oil
Paprika

Flour or bread crumbs
Dash pepper

Cut skin from chicken. Brush each piece with oil. Roll lightly in flour or bread crumbs. Season with pepper and paprika. Bake at 425° for 35 to 40 minutes. Turn and bake 10 to 25 minutes longer or until tender.

FLOUNDER BAKED WITH HOLLANDAISE

1 lb. fresh broccoli spears,
  cooked in unsalted water
4 flounder fillets

½ C. Special Hollandaise Sauce
  (see substitution chart)
Paprika

In greased 13x9x2" baking dish, arrange broccoli spears and top with flounder fillets. Pour Hollandaise Sauce over fillets and sprinkle with paprika. Bake at 350° for 15 to 20 minutes or until fish flakes easily when tested with fork. Serve immediately.

FROZEN BEEF CUBES

6 lbs. beef stew meat
¼ C. vegetable oil
¾ T. salt

1 tsp. pepper
1 qt. hot water

Trim all fat from beef. Brown beef in hot oil in heavy pot. Add salt, pepper and hot water. Cover tightly and simmer 1 to 2 hours or until barely tender. Cool, remove fat and freeze. Allow about ½ cup per person. The above prepared frozen beef cubes could be used in making beef stew.

ITALIAN SPAGHETTI

1½ lbs. ground beef
1½ tsp. salt
½ tsp. basil
¼ tsp. pepper
1 tsp. oregano
2 T. chopped parsley

¼ tsp. anise seed
¼ C. chopped onion
1 clove minced garlic
¼ C. water
1-#2½ can tomatoes
2-6 oz. cans tomato paste

Brown ground beef and onions in small amount of oil and drain. Add remaining ingredients and simmer uncovered, stirring occasionally, until thick, 45 minutes to 1 hour. Serve over hot cooked spaghetti.

LOW CHOLESTEROL CHICKEN POT PIE

½ C. diced carrots
¼ C. diced celery
¼ C. chopped white onion
Chicken broth
1½ C. cooked chicken
⅛ tsp. pepper

3 C. cream of chicken soup
½ C. fresh snow peas
½ C. thinly sliced fresh
  mushrooms
1 recipe double pie crust,
  made with oil

In small amount of chicken broth, saute carrots, celery and onion. Add chicken, soup, remaining vegetables and seasoning; set aside. Roll out pastry dough. Line 1-9" pie pan with ½ of the dough. Fill with chicken filling. Adjust top crust. Tuck edges under and flute. Cut steam holes. Bake at 400° for 20 minutes or until lightly browned.

MEATBALLS IN SPICY YOGURT SAUCE

1 lb. ground raw turkey
1/3 C. finely chopped onion
1/4 C. dry bread crumbs
1 C. lowfat yogurt, divided
1 egg white
1 T. dried parsley flakes

1/2 tsp. ground cumin
1/4 tsp. pepper
1 1/2 tsp. cornstarch
1/2 C. bottled salsa or taco
  sauce
1 tsp. chili powder, optional

Combine turkey, onion, bread crumbs, 1/4 cup yogurt, egg white, parsley, cumin and pepper until blended. Shape into 1" balls (about 30); arrange in circular pattern in 10" glass pie plate. Cover with waxed paper. Microwave on high 4 minutes; rearrange. Microwave 2 minutes or until no longer pink; drain well and set aside. Combine remaining yogurt, cornstarch, salsa and chili powder in a 2-cup microproof measure or bowl. Microwave on medium (70%) power 3 minutes or until mixture boils and is thickened. Whisk after 2 minutes. Pour over meatballs. Microwave, covered with wax paper for 1 minute.   48

MEAT LOAF- CALIFORNIA STYLE

1 lb. ground round of beef
1 C. corn flakes
2 egg whites
¾ tsp. salt
⅛ tsp. pepper

⅓ C. instant dry milk
½ C. water
¼ C. catsup
1 T. Worcestershire sauce
1 C. raisins

Mix the ground round, corn flakes, egg white, salt, pepper, instant dry milk, water, catsup, Worcestershire sauce and raisins. Blend thoroughly. Form into a loaf and place it in a shallow pan. Bake the loaf in a preheated moderate oven (350°) for 1 hour or until loaf is browned.

OMELET

3 egg whites
¼ C. dry cottage cheese

⅛ tsp. salt
1 T. margarine

Beat the egg whites until stiff but not dry. Stir in the cottage cheese and salt. Melt the margarine in an 8" skillet. Pour the egg mixture into it. Bake in a preheated 400° oven 10 minutes or until puffed and delicately browned. Serves 1.

ONION SOUP MEAT LOAF

2 lbs. ground round of beef
½ pkg. dehydrated onion soup
2 egg whites

2 C. cracker crumbs
1 C. hot water

Blend the ground beef, dehydrated onion soup, egg whites, cracker crumbs and water. Mix well, form loaf and place it in a shallow pan. Bake the loaf in a preheated moderate over (350°) for 1¼ hours or until browned. Serves 6 to 8.

ORANGE GLAZED TURKEY

1 lb. breast of turkey
¼ C. orange marmalade

2 T. Dijon mustard
1 T. brown sugar

Cut turkey into 4-½" slices. Make glaze by combining remaining ingredients in small bowl. Heat turkey over hot coals in covered grill, 8 to 10 minutes, turning once and brushing occasionally with glaze.

OVEN-FRIED FILLETS OR STEAKS

2 lbs. fresh or frozen steaks
  or fillets
½ C. reconstituted instant
  dry milk

¾ tsp. salt
1 ½ C. corn flake crumbs or
  toasted dry bread crumbs
¼ C. vegetable oil

Thaw frozen fish. Cut fish into 6 portions. Mix milk and salt. Dip fish in milk and roll in crumbs. Put fish, single layer, skin side down on a well greased baking pan. Pour oil over fish and bake in a preheated very hot oven (500°) for 10 to 15 minutes or until fish are brown and flake easily when tested with a fork.

PAPER BAG CHICKEN

2½ lb. whole fryer
¼ tsp. salt

1 tsp. poultry seasoning
1 brown paper bag

Remove all the visible fat from chicken. Sprinkle the inside of the chicken with salt. Sprinkle the outside of the chicken with poultry seasoning. Put chicken in a brown paper bag and tie it with a string, leaving the bag loose around the chicken. Place the bag in a shallow baking pan and bake it in a preheated slow oven (300°) for 2 hours.

NOTE: Recycled paper bags don't work. Use parchment paper instead.

PEPPERED MEATBALLS AND SPAGHETTI SQUASH

In a medium mixing bowl combine 1 egg white and ¼ cup milk. Stir in 3 tablespoons fine dry bread crumbs, 2 tablespoons chopped green onion and ¼ teaspoon pepper. Add 1 pound lean ground beef; mix well. Shape into 32-1" meatballs. Place on rack in shallow baking pan. Bake in 375° oven for 25 to 30 minutes. Meanwhile, halve 1-3 pound spaghetti squash lengthwise and discard seeds. Place in a Dutch oven. Add water to depth of 2". Bring to boiling; reduce heat. Cover; simmer 25 to 30 minutes. Cook 1½ cups loose-pack frozen mixed cauliflower, broccoli and carrots according to package directions; drain. Halve any large pieces. Combine 1-15½ ounce jar meatless chunky-style spaghetti sauce and 3 tablespoons dry red wine; heat through, stirring occasionally. Gently stir in meatballs and vegetables; heat through. Drain squash. Use a fork to shred pulp onto 4 plates. Top with sauce and grated Parmesan cheese, if desired. Makes 4 servings.

SALMON FUSILLI

A lowfat, cholesterol-fighting meal.

6 oz. fusilli or fettuccine
2 C. broccoli flowerets
1-12½ oz. can boneless,
  skinless pink salmon
1 T. margarine
4 tsp. cornstarch

1 C. skim milk
½ tsp. instant chicken
  bouillon granules
¼ tsp. dried tarragon,
  crushed
1 T. lemon juice

In a kettle cook pasta and broccoli 10 to 12 minutes. Drain. Add drained salmon. In saucepan melt margarine. Blend in cornstarch. Add milk, bouillon and tarragon. Cook until bubbly. Cook 1 minute more. Remove from heat. Stir in lemon juice. Spoon sauce over pasta. Sprinkle with snipped parsley and pepper. Makes 4 servings.

SALMON PATTIES

1-15½ oz. can pink salmon   ½ C. flour
2 egg whites   1½ tsp. baking powder

Drain salmon; set aside 2 tablespoons of the juice. Mix salmon and egg whites until sticky. Stir in flour. Add baking powder to salmon juice; stir into salmon mixture. Form into small patties and fry until golden brown in hot special oil.

STRAW AND HAY

3 oz. linguine for fettuccine
3 oz. green linguine or
  fettuccine
1 C. sliced fresh mushrooms
½ C. frozen peas
¼ C. sliced green onion
1 C. skim milk

1 T. cornstarch
¼ tsp. salt
⅛ tsp. ground nutmeg
⅛ tsp. pepper
¼ C. grated Parmesan
  cheese
¼ C. (2 oz.) finely chopped,
  fully cooked turkey

In a large kettle or Dutch oven bring 2 quarts water to rolling boil. Add pastas. Cook, uncovered, for 8 minutes. Add mushrooms, peas and green onion. Cook for 4 to 5 minutes more or until pasta is tender and vegetables are just tender. Drain well. Meanwhile, for cheese sauce, in a saucepan combine milk, cornstarch, salt, nutmeg and pepper. Cook and stir until thickened and bubbly. Cook and stir 2 minutes more. Add Parmesan cheese and turkey. Combine pasta mixture and cheese sauce. Toss to coat. Makes 6 side-dish servings.

TENDER SWISS STEAK

1 lb. extra-lean round steak   1 onion, cut into rings
¼ C. flour   ¼ C. red wine
Dash of pepper   1-1 lb. can tomatoes

Shake meat in bag with flour and pepper. Brown onion and meat on both sides in wine. Drain to remove any excess fat. Stir in tomatoes. Cover tightly and cook slowly for 1½ to 2 hours until tender.

TROUT AND WINE BAKE

½ C. dry white wine
1 tsp. dried tarragon leaves
8 trout, about 5 to 6 oz. each
4 tsp. lemon juice

Salt, to taste
White pepper
¼ C. melted margarine
½ tsp. chopped parsley

Heat oven to 375°. Brush inside of fish with salt, pepper and melted margarine. Sprinkle with lemon juice, tarragon, salt and white pepper on outside. Pour wine around fish. Cover and bake 15 minutes or until flaky.

TURKEY BARBECUE

1 turkey
Sage
Pepper
Garlic powder

2 stalks celery, chopped
1 lg. onion, chopped
Safflower oil

Wash turkey well. Rub sage, pepper and garlic powder inside cavity. Place celery and onions inside cavity. Skewer neck skin to back; tuck wing tips behind shoulder joints. Rub outside of turkey with safflower oil. Place 25 briquets on each side of barbecue kettle. When coals are ready put in drip pan. Put turkey in roast holder position on grill. Every hour add 8 briquets per side. For a 12-pound turkey allow 2½ hours cooking time; allow 11 minutes per pound for a 20-pound turkey.

TURKEY BURGER

1 lb. lean ground turkey breast
¼ C. oat-bran cereal
1 lg. minced garlic clove
¼ C. finely chopped onion

⅛ C. finely chopped
  green pepper
1 tsp. salt or sodium
  alternative seasoning

Mix all ingredients and form into 4 patties; grill indoors or out on the barbecue. Serve on a toasted bun or choose sourdough bread for less fat and cholesterol.

VEAL ROAST

1 lean veal shoulder, loin or rack of veal roast	Pinch of thyme
2 tsp. olive oil	Garlic powder, to taste
Juice of ½ lemon	Black pepper, to taste
	Pinch of salt

Let meat stand at room temperature for 1 hour; rub with olive oil. Sprinkle with lemon juice and season with thyme, garlic powder, salt and black pepper. Put fat side up on rack in roasting pan. Insert a meat thermometer into thickest part of meat. Bake, uncovered at 425°. Cover loosely with foil. Roast for 15 to 20 minutes per pound; meat thermometer should register 170°.

VEGETABLE MEDLEY QUICHE

1 T. margarine
1 sm. zucchini, sliced
1 sm. green pepper, cut
 in strips
1 sm. red pepper, cut in strips
Low cholesterol pastry crust

1-8 oz. carton egg substitute
1 C. skim milk
¼ tsp. basil leaves
⅛ tsp. ground black pepper

In medium skillet, over medium heat, melt margarine. Add zucchini and pepper; cook, stirring occasionally until tender-crisp. In a medium bowl, mix egg substitute, milk, basil, pepper and vegetables. Spoon mixture into pastry crust and bake at 350° for 40 minutes.

WHITEFISH IN FOIL

2 lbs. fresh or frozen whitefish
    fillets
1 C. sliced fresh green peppers
½ C. thinly sliced onions
⅛ tsp. pepper

¼ C. vegetable oil
2 T. lemon juice
1½ tsp. salt
1 tsp. paprika

Thaw frozen fish. Cut the fish into serving size portions. Cut 6 pieces of heavy duty aluminum foil 12x12". Grease foil lightly. Place a portion of fish skin side down on each portion of foil. Top each portion of fish with 1/6 of the green peppers and onions. Mix oil, lemon juice, salt, paprika and pepper to form a sauce. Pour the sauce over the fish. Bring the foil up over the fish and close all edges with tight double folds. Make 6 packages. Arrange packages on a grill about 5" from moderately hot coals. Cook for 45 to 60 minutes or until fish flakes easily when tested with a fork. Serve hot. Or place the packages in preheated moderate oven (350°) for about 25 minutes, or until fish flakes easily when tested with a fork. Serve an additional packet to each person.   65

YOGURT CHICKEN

1 C. lowfat plain yogurt
2 cloves garlic, minced
1 tsp. ground coriander
½ tsp. hot pepper sauce
Few grains ground black
  pepper
½ tsp. dry mustard

¼ tsp. salt, optional
1 tsp. fresh grated ginger root
3 T. vinegar
1 T. sherry wine
2½ to 3 lb. chicken, cut up
  and skinned
Paprika

Combine yogurt, garlic, seasonings, vinegar and wine in an 8x12" microproof baking dish. Coat chicken parts with yogurt mixture, arranging thicker parts of chicken towards outside of dish. Marinate overnight, turning chicken over once. Sprinkle with paprika. Microwave, covered, with waxed paper on high 20 minutes or until meat near the bone is no longer pink and the juices run clear, rotating dish once. Let stand, covered, for 10 minutes before serving. Serves 4.

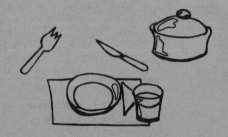

VEGETABLES

AROMATIC VEGETABLE CASSEROLE

1 C. onions, sliced
2 C. celery, sliced in 1½"
  pieces
2 C. or 1 can whole tomatoes
  and juice
1½ C. carrots, sliced
¾ C. green peppers, sliced

1 can yellow beans
1 can green beans
4 T. margarine
3 T. Minute tapioca
¼ tsp. pepper
Salt to taste

Combine all ingredients and pour into large casserole dish and bake for 1½ hours in a 350° oven.

ASPARAGUS IN MARINADE

¼ C. oil
2 T. white wine vinegar
¼ tsp. salt
¼ tsp. dry mustard

10½ oz. can cut spears
 asparagus, drained
1 T. chopped green
 bell pepper
1 T. chopped red bell pepper
1 T. sliced green onion

In small jar with tight-fitting lid, combine oil, vinegar, salt and dry mustard; shake well. Arrange asparagus in small shallow dish. Sprinkle with peppers and onion; pour dressing over asparagus. Cover; refrigerate at least 30 minutes to blend flavors. Serves 3 (½-cup each).

BAKED CARROTS

1 T. margarine
2 T. chopped onion
1 lb. carrots, sliced and
    cooked
1 C. skim milk

¾ C. egg substitute
2 T. chopped parsley
½ tsp. ground nutmeg
⅛ tsp. ground black pepper

In small skillet over medium heat, melt margarine. Add onion and cook, stirring occasionally, until tender. Remove from heat. In electric blender or food processor container, blend carrots, skim milk and egg substitute until mixture is smooth. Stir in onion mixture, parsley, nutmeg and pepper. Pour into sprayed 1-quart casserole. Bake at 350° at 45 to 50 minutes. Serve hot.

BASIC FRIED RICE

1 ½ C. water
¾ tsp. salt
1 C. raw rice
2 T. oil

½ C. chopped green onions
¼ tsp. minced garlic
2 T. low sodium soy sauce

Bring the water and salt to a boil. Stir in the rice, bring to a boil again, cover and cook over low heat 15 minutes or until the rice is tender and dry. Chill. Heat the oil in a skillet; stir the rice into it until coated. Mix in the onions and garlic; cook 3 minutes. Blend in the soy sauce. Serves 6.

BROWNED OVEN POTATOES

Steam whole until barely done 4 medium-size potatoes. Remove skins and place potatoes in a small flat pan. Dissolve 2 vegetable bouillon cubes (or fat free meat drippings) in ½ cup boiling water, 1 tablespoon oil. Pour over potatoes. Sprinkle with paprika if desired. Brown in a hot oven (400°) for about 30 minutes. Add water if needed. For added browning, place under the broiler 1 to 2 minutes. Serves 4.

CORN SAUTE

1 T. margarine
12 oz. can whole kernel corn
  with sweet peppers, drained

1 T. chopped green onion,
  including top

In medium skillet over medium-high heat, melt margarine. Add corn and onion; saute until thoroughly heated. Serves 3 (½-cup each).

For Microwave: Place margarine in 1-quart microwave-safe casserole. Microwave on high for 15 to 30 seconds or until margarine is melted. Add corn and onion. Cover; microwave on high for 3 to 4½ minutes or until thoroughly heated, stirring once during cooking.

DILLED POTATO SALAD WITH PEAS

3 lbs. sm. red new potatoes
1-11 oz. pkg. frozen peas

1/3 C. light mayonnaise
2 T. lemon juice
1 to 2 cloves garlic, minced
1/2 tsp. salt, optional

1/4 C. green onion slices
1 C. plain lowfat yogurt

1 to 2 T. snipped fresh dill or
 2 tsp. dried dill
1/2 tsp. sage
1/4 tsp. pepper

Wash new potatoes, cut into 1/4" slices and cook in large saucepan with boiling water to cover. Boil gently 10 minutes or until potatoes are just tender. Do not overcook. Drain and cool. Meanwhile, cook frozen peas 2 minutes in boiling water. Drain and cool. Combine yogurt, mayonnaise, lemon juice, garlic, dill, sage, salt (if used) and pepper; mix until smooth. Combine with potatoes, peas and onion slices. Toss gently. Chill 1 to 3 hours before serving. Makes 10 servings.

EGGPLANT BARBECUED

1 med. eggplant, unpeeled
⅓ C. olive oil
2 T. tarragon white wine
  vinegar

1 clove garlic, minced
⅛ tsp. or less salt
¼ tsp. oregano

Slice eggplant lengthwise into 8 wedges. Mix oil, vinegar, garlic, salt and oregano in a covered container and shake. Pour over eggplant. Drain excess oil. Grill eggplant slices over hot coals until tender, turning once.

GLAZED GINGERED CARROTS

1 lb. carrots, peeled and cut
  in ¼" slices
1 T. special margarine

¾ T. sugar
1 tsp. ginger
2 T. fresh parsley

Steam carrots until tender. In frying pan, melt margarine. Add carrots and toss. Sprinkle with sugar and ginger. Mix lightly to coat carrots and continue cooking until carrots are lightly glazed, about 1 to 2 minutes. Add parsley.

GLAZED ONIONS

¾ lb. sm. white onions
2 T. margarine

1 tsp. sugar
¼ tsp. salt

Peel onions and cover with water. Bring to a boil. Cook over low heat until barely tender; drain. Melt the margarine in a skillet. Add the onions, sugar and salt; cover and cook over low heat until onions are glazed, shaking the pan frequently.

GRANDMA'S BAKED BEANS

1 lb. beans
Water for soaking beans
½ tsp. salt
¼ C. brown sugar, packed

¼ C. molasses
1 tsp. dry mustard
1 sm. onion, chopped

Wash the beans, place in a kettle, cover with cold water and soak overnight. Pour off the water and replace it with fresh water. Bring the beans to the boil, reduce heat and simmer for about 90 minutes. Drain the beans, reserving the liquid. Place the beans in a bean pot. Combine the salt, sugar, molasses, mustard and onion with ½ cup of the cooking liquid. Pour over the beans. If necessary, pour on additional cooking liquid until the beans are just covered. Cover the bean pot and put it in a 300° oven for 8 hours. The beans should be covered with liquid for the first 7 hours, so add more cooking liquid as needed.

HARVARD BEETS

Wash, cook, remove the skins and cut into thin slices or cubes 6 large beets. Mix together ½ cup sugar, 1 tablespoon cornstarch and ½ teaspoon salt. Add ½ cup vinegar. Cook 5 minutes, stirring constantly. Pour the boiling liquid over the beets and let stand a few minutes before serving. Serves 6.

HARVEST BEANS

2 C. frozen cut green beans
  or cut fresh green beans
¼ C. water
3 T. sliced green onions

½ tsp. chicken flavor instant
  bouillon
⅛ to ¼ tsp. cinnamon
Dash pepper
2 T. catsup

In medium saucepan, combine all ingredients except catsup. Bring to a boil; reduce heat. Simmer uncovered 8 to 10 minutes or until beans are tender. Stir in catsup. Serves 4 (½-cup each).

For Microwave: In 1-quart microwave-safe bowl or dish, combine beans, 3 tablespoons water and remaining ingredients except catsup; cover. Microwave on high for 9 to 12 minutes or until beans are tender. Stir in catsup.

HASH BROWNS

1 potato per person
½ tsp. onion per potato,
  optional
Dash pepper

½ tsp. safflower oil
  per potato
Pinch of salt, if desired

Steam potatoes in their skins. Chill, peel and shred. Mix with onion, oil, salt
and pepper. Make into thin patties. Brown in a Teflon skillet over medium
heat 10 to 12 minutes. Turn. Brown 8 to 10 minutes longer or to desired
brownness.

HOT POTATO SALAD

2 qts. cold, sliced, boiled
  potatoes
6 T. vegetable oil
3 T. white vinegar
3 T. lemon juice

2 T. finely chopped onion
1 tsp. salt
¼ tsp. pepper
3 T. chopped parsley
3 T. imitation bacon bits

Layer potatoes in 3-quart greased casserole. Mix the oil, vinegar, lemon juice, onions, salt and pepper and heat to simmering. Remove the oil mixture from the heat and pour it over the potatoes. Sprinkle the salad with the parsley and imitation bacon bits and heat it in moderate oven (350°) for about 30 minutes or until hot. Gently stir the salad and serve hot.

ITALIAN GREEN BEANS

3 T. oil
½ C. chopped onions
1 clove garlic, minced
1-20 oz. can tomatoes,
  drained
¼ tsp. salt

¼ tsp. freshly ground
  black pepper
¼ tsp. oregano
1 bay leaf
2 lbs. green beans or 3 pkgs.
  frozen

Saute onions in saucepan with oil. Add the garlic, tomatoes, salt, pepper, oregano and bay leaf, bring to a boil and cook over low heat 20 minutes. Add the fresh or frozen beans to the tomato mixture. Cover and cook over low heat 30 minutes.

MAKE YOUR OWN POTATO CHIPS

1 potato per person   *Safflower or corn oil*

Cut potatoes crosswise into paper-thin rounds; brush with safflower oil.
Bake on baking sheet at 425° for 20 minutes. Turn, bake 15 to 20 minutes or
until brown.

MARINATED VEGETABLES

1 C. corn oil
1 C. cider vinegar
⅓ C. sugar
1 tsp. salt or less
½ tsp. pepper
2-16 oz. cans red kidney
  beans, drained

2-16 oz. cans whole baby
  carrots, drained
½ C. finely chopped onion
3-10 oz. pkgs. frozen broccoli
  spears, cooked and drained

Mix first 5 ingredients. Place beans and carrots in 13x9x2'' dish. Sprinkle with onion. Top with broccoli. Pour oil mixture over vegetables. Cover and refrigerate overnight. Drain and arrange on platter. Makes 12 servings. Wait a day for flavor to develop.

MASHED CARROTS

Wash, scrape, cut into small pieces and cook until tender 10 medium-size carrots. When cooked, put through a ricer or mash. Add warm skim milk to moisten (about ¼ cup), ½ teaspoon salt and dash of pepper. Serve at once. Serves 6.

VARIATION: Form nests of mashed carrots and fill with cooked peas.

MASHED POTATOES

Cook in their jackets until tender 4 large potatoes. Remove skins and mash the potatoes. Blend or shake together in a covered jar until smooth:

1 T. vegetable oil
½ C. potato cooking water
⅓ C. skim milk powder

1 tsp. salt
Pepper, to taste

Heat and beat into the mashed potatoes. Add hot potato cooking water if more moisture is needed to make the potatoes light and fluffy. Serve at once. Sprinkle with Butter Buds. Serves 6.

MINTED PEAS

17 oz. can peas, undrained   1 tsp. mint flakes, crushed
1 tsp. margarine

Place peas in medium saucepan. Bring to a boil. Reduce heat; simmer 1 minute. Drain. Stir in mint and margarine. Serves 4 (½-cup each).
For Microwave: Place peas in 1-quart microwave-safe dish; cover. Microwave on high for 2½ to 3½ minutes or until thoroughly heated. Drain. Stir in mint and margarine.

MIXED VEGETABLE GOULASH

2 T. oil
¾ C. thinly sliced onions
1 C. diced green peppers
1-20 oz. can tomatoes
1 C. diced potatoes
2 pkgs. frozen mixed
  vegetables, thawed

1 tsp. salt
¼ tsp. freshly ground
  black pepper
1 tsp. paprika
1 tsp. sugar
1 T. flour
2 T. water

Heat the oil in a casserole; saute the onions 5 minutes. Add the green peppers; saute 5 minutes. Stir in tomatoes, potatoes, mixed vegetables, salt, pepper, paprika and sugar. Bring to a boil and cook over low heat 20 minutes. Mix together flour and water; stir into the vegetables until thickened.

MUSHROOMS AND PEAS

Shell enough peas to make 2 cups of peas (or use 2 packages frozen peas). Wipe, trim and slice ½ pound fresh mushrooms. Simmer peas and mushrooms in 1 cup skim milk and ½ teaspoon salt. When peas are tender, thicken liquid with 2 to 3 teaspoons cornstarch, mixed with a little water. Stir gently until cornstarch is cooked. Serve in sauce dishes with sauce. Sauce may be omitted. Drain peas and mushrooms and save the liquid for soup. Serves 6.

OVEN FRENCH FRIES

Peel and cut into French-fry size 4 medium-size potatoes. Remove all excess moisture and place the potatoes in a medium-size bowl. Sprinkle with 2 tablespoons vegetable oil. Toss the potatoes as if making a tossed green salad. When the oil and potatoes are thoroughly mixed, spread the potatoes out on a cookie sheet and place in a hot oven (475 to 500°) for 35 minutes. Turn the potatoes so they will brown evenly on both sides. For added browning, place under the broiler 1 to 2 minutes. May sprinkle with salt before serving or a salt substitute. Serves 6.

QUICK BEANS WITH BASIL

1 T. finely chopped onion
1 garlic clove, minced
1 T. margarine
Dash pepper

16 oz. can cut green beans,
  drained
1 tsp. basil leaves

In medium saucepan, saute onion and garlic in margarine until tender. Add beans, basil and pepper; stir well. Cover; cook 2 to 3 minutes or until thoroughly heated. Serves 4 (½-cup each).

For Microwave: In 1-quart microwave-safe casserole or bowl, place onion, garlic and margarine. Microwave on high for 1 to 1½ minutes or until onion is tender. Add beans, basil and pepper; stir well. Cover; microwave on high for 2 to 3 minutes or until thoroughly heated.

RICE IN BROTH

Bring to a boil 2½ cups consomme, bouillon, beef or chicken broth. Add ½ teaspoon salt (or as needed), 1 cup enriched white rice or enriched brown rice. Cover tightly and cook over low heat about 25 minutes. If a drier rice is desired, remove cover and cook 5 minutes longer over low heat. Serves 6.

VARIATION: Substitute 1¼ cups water and 1¼ cups tomato juice or vegetable juice for the broth.

SCALLOPED POTATOES

3 T. margarine
2 T. all-purpose flour
2 C. skim milk
¼ tsp. pepper
½ C. chopped onion

⅛ tsp. onion powder
⅛ tsp. garlic powder
5 med. potatoes, thinly sliced

Melt margarine in a saucepan. Add flour and mix well. Gradually add milk while stirring constantly. Cook over medium heat, stirring until thickened. Add pepper, onion powder and garlic powder. Place potatoes and chopped onion in a lightly-oiled 1½-quart casserole, add sauce and mix. Cover and bake in 350° oven 30 minutes. Stir gently and bake uncovered an additional 30 to 40 minutes or until lightly browned and potatoes are tender. Serves 5.

SPANISH RICE

1 med. onion, chopped	1 C. uncooked long grain
1 sm. green pepper, chopped	white rice
1 clove garlic, minced	½ tsp. seasoned salt
1 T. vegetable or olive oil	⅛ tsp. pepper
1-16 oz. can tomatoes	¼ tsp. chili powder
	¼ tsp. cumin

In a 2-quart casserole, combine onion, green pepper, garlic and oil. Microwave covered, on high for 2 to 3 minutes or until tender. Drain tomatoes, reserving liquid and chopping tomatoes. Add enough water to reserved liquid to make 2 cups. Add to onion mixture with tomatoes, rice and seasoning. Microwave, covered, on high for 5 minutes or until boiling. Microwave on medium-low (30%) for 14 to 16 minutes or until rice is tender. Let stand, covered, 5 minutes. Serves 6.

SQUASH CASSEROLE

yum!

1 lg. butternut squash
3 to 4 tomatoes
1 lg. sweet onion
1 lg. fresh green pepper

¼ C. margarine
Salt and pepper, optional
½ to 1 tsp. leaf oregano

Slice vegetables. Place half of the squash in a well greased casserole. Cover with the sliced tomatoes, onions and green peppers. Dot with margarine and sprinkle with salt, pepper and oregano. Add the remaining squash to casserole, sprinkle it with seasonings and dot it with the remaining margarine. Cover the casserole tightly and bake it in a preheated moderate (350°) oven for 45 minutes. Remove the cover of casserole and continue to bake for about 30 minutes or until squash is tender and lightly browned.

SWEET-SOUR BEETS

2-16 oz. cans sliced beets,
   drained
1 sm. onion, thinly sliced,
   separated into rings

⅓ C. cider vinegar
¼ C. oil
½ C. sugar
¼ tsp. salt

In medium non-metal bowl, combine beets and onion. In small jar with tight-fitting lid, combine vinegar, oil, sugar and salt; shake well. Pour over beets. Refrigerate at least 1 hour to blend flavors. Makes 6 (½-cup each) servings.

TEMPTING CARROTS

4 C. carrots, cut into 1"
  pieces
¾ C. green onions, cut
  into 1" pieces

¼ C. margarine
2 T. honey
¼ to ½ tsp. salt

In medium saucepan, cook carrots in boiling water until tender, about 7 to 9 minutes. Add onions; cook 2 minutes. Drain well. Stir in margarine, honey and salt; heat thoroughly. Serves 8 (½-cup each).

For Microwave: In 1½-quart microwave-safe casserole or bowl, place carrots and 2 tablespoons water; cover. Microwave on high for 9 to 11 minutes or until tender, stirring once during cooking. Add onions; cover. Microwave on high for 1 to 1½ minutes or until onions are crisp-tender; drain. Stir in margarine, honey and salt. Microwave on high for 30 to 60 seconds or until thoroughly heated, stirring once during cooking.

TIP: Baby carrots can be substituted for carrot pieces.

TWICE BAKED POTATOES WITH COTTAGE CHEESE

4 med. potatoes, baked
1 C. lowfat cottage cheese
½ C. lowfat milk

1 T. minced onion
Freshly ground black pepper
Paprika
Dried parsley flakes

Cut hot potatoes in half lengthwise. Scoop out potatoes, leaving skins intact for restuffing. With wire whisk, beat potatoes with cottage cheese, milk and onion. Spoon mixture back into skins. Sprinkle with paprika and parsley flakes and black pepper. Bake 10 minutes.

WESTERN STYLE BROCCOLI

2 T. lemon juice
¼ tsp. pepper
¼ tsp. oregano
¼ tsp. garlic clove

¼ C. oil
1-10 oz. pkg. frozen or 1 lb.
  fresh broccoli

Mix all ingredients together, except broccoli. Let stand for 30 minutes. Cook frozen broccoli according to directions on package. If using fresh broccoli, wash, trim, cut into small stalks and cook in boiling unsalted water for 10 to 15 minutes or until tender but still crisp. Remove garlic from dressing, stir well and pour over hot broccoli just before serving. Serves 3.

NOTES • NOTES • NOTES • NOTES • NOTES

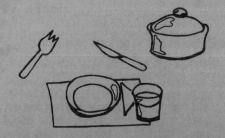

SALADS

BROCCOLI SALAD

1 pkg. lemon gelatin
½ tsp. salt
1 C. boiling water
1-10 oz. pkg. chopped
  broccoli, cut into small
  cubes

2 tsp. minced onion
½ C. lowfat cottage cheese
2 T. reduced calorie
  mayonnaise
2 tsp. prepared mustard

Completely dissolve gelatin and salt in boiling water. Add broccoli and onion; stir until broccoli thaws and separates. Add lowfat cottage cheese, mayonnaise and mustard. Pour into individual dishes or a bowl. Chill until set, at least 30 minutes.

101

CARROT AND PINEAPPLE SALAD

2 C. shredded fresh carrots
½ C. raisins
¼ C. miniature marshmallows

1 C. drained crushed pineapple
½ C. low calorie mayonnaise

Mix all ingredients together and chill before serving. Serves 4 to 6.

CHICKEN SALAD

3 C. diced, cooked chicken
1½ C. chopped celery
½ C. chopped English walnuts

2 T. lemon juice
¼ tsp. salt
¼ tsp. white pepper
1 C. low calorie mayonnaise

Mix the chicken, celery, walnuts, lemon juice, salt and pepper. Toss the salad gently. Add the mayonnaise and mix lightly. Refrigerate until chilled.

COTTAGE CHEESE SALAD

Slice as thin as possible 8 medium radishes and 1 small cucumber. Chop very fine 4 scallions (both the white and green parts). Add the mixture to 2 cups skim milk cottage cheese. Mix together well and add salt to taste. Serve chilled on leaf of lettuce. Serves 4.

ITALIAN LIMA BEAN SALAD

Cook until tender, drain and rinse in cold water (save cooking water for soups or sauces) 2 cups green lima beans.

MIX TOGETHER:
4 T. oil
1½ to 2 T. wine vinegar
2 T. chopped onion
Pepper

2 T. chopped parsley
1 garlic bud, finely chopped
Salt

Mix the dressing thoroughly through the beans and chill. Serve on crisp greens surrounded by 12 slices tomato garnished with 12 slices green pepper. Serves 6.

JOAN'S APPLE JELLO SALAD

3 sm. boxes strawberry jello
2 med. apples, peeled and
 grated

1½ C. crushed pineapple,
 drained

Dissolve jello in 3 cups boiling water. Use pineapple juice and enough cold water to make the 3 cups. Add pineapple and apples to jello mixture and stir occasionally until it starts to set.

ORIENTAL NOODLE SALAD

1 lb. fresh noodles, Chinese-style
1-8 oz. container plain yogurt
2 T. soy sauce
4 green onions with tops, sliced diagonally
1½ tsp. Dijon-style mustard
Salt and pepper, to taste
1 C. shredded carrot
6 oz. fresh, blanched snow peas or 1-6 oz. pkg. frozen snow peas, thawed
1 to 2 T. toasted sesame seeds

Cook noodles in boiling water for 2 minutes, or until al dente. Drain immediately and rinse under cold water until noodles are room temperature; drain. Combine yogurt, soy sauce, green onion, mustard, salt and pepper in large bowl. Add noodles and carrots, tossing to coat evenly. To serve, arrange noodle mixture on platter; top with snow peas. Sprinkle with sesame seeds. Makes 8 servings.

PEAR AND RED GRAPE SALAD

3 C. torn spinach leaves
1 med. pear, sliced
1 C. seedless red grapes
½ C. sliced celery
¼ C. pecan pieces
½ C. Lemon Honey Dressing

Place spinach leaves on large platter. Arrange pear, grapes, celery and pecans decoratively on top. Drizzle with ½ of dressing. Serve with remaining dressing. Makes 4 servings.

LEMON HONEY DRESSING:
¼ C. lemon juice
2 T. special oil
2 T. honey

In container with lid, combine all dressing ingredients. Shake well. Cover and refrigerate to blend flavors. Store in refrigerator. Makes ½ cup.

PINEAPPLE-CARROT MOLDED SALAD

Drain juice from ½ cup crushed pineapple. Use juice with sufficient water to prepare 1 package lime or lemon gelatin. When cool but not firm, add the drained pineapple and ½ cup grated carrots, 1 tablespoon vinegar and ¼ teaspoon salt. Pour into a mold and chill until firm. Unmold on crisp greens. Serves 4.

PINEAPPLE-GRAPEFRUIT SALAD

Drain and mix juice from ½ cup unsweetened grapefruit broken into bite-size pieces, ¾ cup unsweetened pineapple tidbits. Prepare according to package directions 1 package lemon gelatin using 1 cup juice mixture. Mix together and reserve for topping 2 tablespoons juice mixture and ¾ cup skim milk cottage cheese. Cool gelatin and stir in 1 cup skim milk cottage cheese. Arrange drained fruit in individual molds or a single large mold. Pour the gelatin mixture over the fruit. Place in the refrigerator to set. To serve, unmold on crisp lettuce and put 1 tablespoon of the reserved skim milk cottage cheese on top of each serving. Needs no added dressing. Serves 6.

TOMATO ASPIC SALAD

HEAT TOGETHER:
1¾ C. tomato juice
¼ tsp. salt

⅛ tsp. pepper
1 bay leaf

REMOVE BAY LEAF AND ADD:
½ tsp. paprika
1 T. onion juice

1 tsp. lemon juice

SOAK:
1 T. gelatin in ¼ C. cold
* water*

Combine tomato juice and gelatin and cool. Stir in finely chopped ½ cup celery, ¼ cup green onion and 2 tablespoons parsley. Pour into individual molds and place in refrigerator to set. Serves 6.

TURKEY-APPLE SALAD

1 can chunk white turkey,
  drained
¾ C. chopped apple
½ C. sliced celery

2 T. raisins
⅓ C. prepared Italian dressing
1 T. brown sugar

In medium bowl, gently stir together chunk turkey, apple, celery and raisins. In cup, stir together dressing and brown sugar; pour over turkey mixture. Toss gently to coat. Serve on lettuce leaves. Makes 1½ cups or 2 servings.

WALDORF SALAD

PREPARE:
1 C. cubed apples　　　*½ C. sliced bananas*
¼ C. diced celery　　　*¼ C. pitted and diced dates*

Soak the fruit 30 minutes in ½ cup orange or pineapple juice. Serve on crisp lettuce. Serves 4.

YOGURT PASTA TOSS

1½ C. plain lowfat yogurt
½ tsp. each thyme and
  rosemary
⅛ tsp. each salt and pepper
1 lb. turkey sausage (Italian if
  possible, with casing removed)

1 sm. leek, cut into julienne
  strips
8 oz. uncooked linguine
1 C. cooked peas
10 cherry tomatoes, quartered

Combine yogurt and seasonings. Refrigerate, covered, 1 to 2 hours to allow flavors to blend. Meanwhile, cook sausage and leek over medium heat until sausage is brown and crumbly. Drain off excess fat. Cook linguine according to package directions; drain. Combine sausage-leek mixture, peas, tomatoes and pasta. Toss with yogurt mixture. Serve immediately.

YUMMY VEGETABLE SALAD

1-16 oz. can French-style
  green beans, drained
1-16 oz. can white corn,
  drained
1-16 oz. can peas, drained

1 C. chopped celery
1 C. chopped green pepper
¼ c. chopped onion

DRESSING:
¾ C. white vinegar
¾ C. sugar

½ C. vegetable oil
½ to 1 tsp. celery seed

Place celery and green peppers in water and refrigerate overnight. Heat ingredients for dressing over low flame long enough to dissolve sugar. Cool and pour over vegetables. Refrigerate in covered dish overnight. Next morning drain celery and peppers; add to mixture. Serves 15 people.

NOTES • NOTES • NOTES • NOTES • NOTES

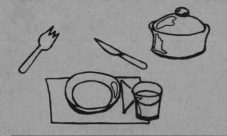

DESSERTS

AMAZING HOT WATER FROSTING

1 egg white
¾ C. sugar
¼ tsp. cream of tartar

1 tsp. vanilla
¼ C. boiling water

Mix the egg white, sugar, cream of tartar and vanilla in a mixer bowl. Start the mixer at high speed and gradually add the boiling water to the egg white mixture. Whip until it stands in peaks and cools.

ANGEL FOOD CAKE

1¾ C. egg whites (12 egg whites)
1¼ C. sifted cake flour
¾ C. sugar
½ tsp. salt

1½ tsp. cream of tartar
1 C. sugar
¾ tsp. almond flavoring
1 tsp. vanilla

Use room temperature egg whites. Sift the flour and ¾ cup sugar together twice. Beat the egg whites with the salt and cream of tartar at a high speed until soft peaks are formed. Add 1 cup sugar gradually, beating it at a high speed to form a meringue. Add the almond flavoring and vanilla to the meringue and mix lightly. Remove the beater from the bowl and add the flour mixture, a quarter at a time, folding it in gently with a wire whisk or rubber scraper. Fold only until the flour mixture is blended into the meringue. Push the batter into an ungreased 10" tube pan. Cut gently through the batter to remove air pockets. Bake in a preheated moderate oven (375°) for 30 to 35 minutes or until the cake springs back when touched in the center. Invert the cake on a funnel and let it hang until it is cold. Carefully loosen the cake from the pan with a spatula and remove it to a plate. Serve plain or frost with a light frosting, if desired.

BANANA CREAM PIE

2¼ C. water
1 C. instant dry milk
¾ C. sugar
2 slightly beaten egg whites
¼ C. cornstarch
¼ tsp. salt'
4 drops yellow food coloring

2 T. margarine
2 tsp. vanilla
2 lg. bananas
1 prebaked 8" pie shell
2 egg whites
¼ tsp. cream of tartar
¼ C. sugar

Mix water, instant dry milk, ¾ cup sugar, 2 egg whites, cornstarch, salt and yellow food coloring in a heavy saucepan. Simmer over a low heat, stirring constantly until thickened. Stir and cook for 2 minutes longer. Remove from heat, add margarine and vanilla; stir lightly until the margarine is melted. Cool and add bananas and pour into the pie shell. Mix 2 egg whites and cream of tartar and beat until frothy. Add ¼ cup sugar gradually and beat at a high speed to form a meringue. Spread the meringue on the pie, being careful to seal the meringue to the edges of the crust so that it will not shrink while baking. Bake the pie in a preheated hot oven (425°) for 8 to 10 minutes or until meringue is lightly browned. Makes 1 pie.

CHERRIES JUBILEE

2 C. pitted Bing cherries,
  with juice
½ C. currant jelly

1 T. cornstarch
1 T. grated orange rind
2 T. heated brandy

Pour juice from cherries into saucepan with the currant jelly, cornstarch and orange rind. Cook over low heat until the jelly melts. Stir into the cherries. Cook and simmer 10 minutes. At the table, pour the warm brandy over the cherries in the serving pan and flame. Spoon into meringue shells or over ice milk while cherries are still flaming. Yield: 8 servings.

CHOCOLATE ICE MILK

1 env. unflavored gelatin
¼ C. water
2 C. skim milk or ½% lowfat
  milk
3 T. unsweetened cocoa

⅓ C. sugar
Pinch of salt
1 T. oil
1 egg white
1 tsp. vanilla

Sprinkle gelatin over water in micro-proof custard cup; let stand 1 minute. Microwave on high 30 seconds or until gelatin dissolves; cool to room temperature. In large bowl combine ¾ cup milk, cocoa, sugar, salt, oil, egg white, vanilla and gelatin mixture. Beat at medium speed with electric mixer until foamy, about 3 minutes. Stir in remaining milk. Pour into shallow metal pan (loaf or 8" square). Place in coldest part of freezer until mixture is almost set, about 20 to 30 minutes, stirring occasionally. Transfer back to large bowl. Beat at medium speed with electric mixer and return to freezer until set.

COCOA BROWNIE CUPCAKES

¾ C. cocoa
2 T. instant dry milk
1½ C. sugar
1½ C. all-purpose flour
½ tsp. baking powder

4 egg whites
1 T. vanilla
⅔ C. vegetable oil
1 C. chopped pecans

Mix the cocoa, instant dry milk, sugar, flour and baking powder together in a mixing bowl. Blend the egg whites, vanilla and vegetable oil and beat with rotary beater until well blended. Add the egg white mixture and nuts to the flour mixture and stir only until well blended (do not beat). Spoon the batter into foil-lined cupcake pans and bake them in a preheated moderate oven (350°) for 30 to 35 minutes.

COCOA FUDGE FROSTING

1 lb. pkg. powdered sugar
½ C. cocoa
1 stick softened margarine

1 tsp. vanilla
2 T. water
¼ C. white syrup

Blend the powdered sugar, cocoa, margarine and vanilla in a mixer bowl. Mix the water and syrup and heat them to simmering, but do not boil. Add the hot syrup to the sugar mixture. Frost a 1-9" layer cake.

DOUBLE CHOCOLATE CREAM PIE

2½ C. water
1 C. instant dry milk
1 C. sugar
2 slightly beaten egg whites
¼ C. cornstarch
¼ tsp. salt
¼ C. cocoa

¼ C. margarine
2 tsp. vanilla
3 egg whites
¼ tsp. cream of tartar
¼ C. sugar
1 T. cocoa
2 T. sugar
1 baked 9" pastry shell

Blend the water, instant dry milk, 1 cup sugar, 2 egg whites, cornstarch, salt, cocoa and margarine in a heavy saucepan. Simmer over a low heat, stirring constantly, until thickened. Stir and cook for 2 minutes longer. Remove the filling from the heat, add the vanilla, cool slightly and pour into the pie shell. Mix 3 egg whites and cream of tartar and beat until frothy. Mix ¼ cup sugar gradually and beat at high speed to form a meringue. Combine 1 tablespoon cocoa and 2 tablespoons sugar, fold into the meringue. Spread the meringue on the pie being careful to seal the edges of the meringue to the edges of the crust so that it will not shrink while baking. Bake in a preheated hot oven (400°) for 8 to 10 minutes or until meringue is lightly browned.

EGGLESS CHOCOLATE CAKE

3 C. flour
2 C. sugar
⅓ C. cocoa
1 tsp. salt
2 tsp. soda

¾ C. oil
2 tsp. vanilla
1 T. vinegar
2 C. water

Sift the first 5 ingredients into the ungreased pan that you will bake in. Mix in the rest of the ingredients with a fork. Mix well and bake at 350° for about 40 minutes. This is a very good moist cake that is rich in chocolate color.

FAVORITE AND EASY PAT-A-PIE OIL PASTRY

Into an 8 or 9" pie plate, sift together 2 cups sifted all-purpose flour, 2 teaspoons sugar and a pinch of salt. With fork, whip together ⅔ cup salad oil and 3 tablespoons milk. Pour over flour mixture. Mix with fork until all flour is dampened. Reserve about ⅓ cup of dough for top crust. Press remaining dough against bottom and sides of pie plate. Crimp edges. For single crust pie, prick sides and bottom with fork and bake at 450° for 10 minutes. May also fill with a fruit filling and sprinkle top with remaining dough. Bake as directed in a fruit pie recipe.

GREAT MARSHMALLOW FROSTING

⅔ C. sugar
½ C. water
1 T. white corn syrup
3 egg whites

1 tsp. cream of tartar
⅓ C. sugar
1 tsp. vanilla

Blend ⅔ cup sugar, water and corn syrup in a heavy saucepan. Stir over a low heat until the sugar is dissolved. Raise the heat and cook without stirring until a few drops form a soft ball in cold water or until it registers 238° on a candy thermometer. Beat the egg whites with the cream of tartar until foamy. Slowly beat ⅓ cup sugar into the egg whites to form a meringue. Beating constantly at high speed, gradually pour the hot syrup over the meringue. Continue beating until the frosting is completely cool and firm. Add vanilla.

LEMON ICE-CREAM DESSERT

2 T. special margarine
1 T. flour
⅛ tsp. salt

3½ C. skim milk
¼ C. sugar
½ C. lemon juice
2 tsp. grated lemon rind

Melt the margarine in a saucepan. Mix in the flour and salt. Slowly add half the milk, stirring steadily to the boiling point. Blend in the sugar, then cook over low heat 5 minutes. Remove from the heat and stir in the remaining milk. Turn into a refrigerator tray and freeze until sides set. Turn into a bowl, add lemon juice and rind; beat until frothy. Return to the tray and freeze until set.

OLD-FASHIONED TAPIOCA PUDDING

⅛ C. egg substitute
1 egg white
3 T. Minute tapioca
⅛ tsp. salt

4 T. sugar
¾ tsp. vanilla
2 C. milk

In saucepan combine egg substitute, milk, tapioca, salt and 3 tablespoons sugar; let stand for 5 minutes. Beat egg whites until foamy; gradually add in remaining sugar. Beat until egg whites form stiff peaks; set aside. Cook tapioca over medium heat, stirring constantly until mixture comes to a full boil, about 6 to 8 minutes. Gradually add into beaten egg whites. Add vanilla and stir enough to mix. Cool for 20 minutes and chill.

PEACH PUDDING DESSERT

1 C. all-purpose flour
C. granulated sugar
2 tsp. baking powder
¼ tsp. salt
½ C. skim milk
3 T. vegetable oil

1-16 oz. can sliced peaches, ¾
  drained
1 C. packed brown sugar
¼ C. finely chopped nuts
1 tsp. ground cinnamon
1 C. boiling water

Heat oven to 350°. Mix flour, granulated sugar, baking powder and salt. Beat in milk and oil until smooth. Pour into ungreased baking pan, 8x8x2". Place peaches on top. Blend brown sugar, nuts and cinnamon; sprinkle over peaches. Pour boiling water on peaches. Bake until wooden pick inserted in center comes out clean, 60 to 70 minutes.

PEANUT BUTTER COOKIES WITH EGG WHITES

4 egg whites
1⅔ C. granulated sugar

2 C. non-hydrogenated
  peanut butter

Beat egg whites until stiff. Set aside. Blend peanut butter and sugar; add in egg whites. Drop by teaspoonfuls onto baking sheets. Flatten slightly with prongs of fork. Bake at 325° for 20 minutes. Cool on wire racks.

PIE CRUST

2 C. flour

½ C. corn oil

4 or 5 T. ice water

1 pinch of salt

Sift together flour and salt. Pour oil and cold water into measuring cup. (Do not stir.) Add all at once to the flour mixture. Stir lightly with fork. Form into 2 balls; flatten dough slightly. Roll each ball between waxed paper or Saran Wrap. Peel off top sheet of paper and fit dough paper side up into pie plate. Remove paper. For a single crust pie, bake at 450° for 10 to 12 minutes, until golden. For a double crust pie, bake at 425° for 20 minutes, then reduce to 375° for 40 minutes.

PUMPKIN CHIFFON PIE

¾ C. brown sugar
1 env. unflavored gelatin
¼ tsp. salt
1 tsp. cinnamon
½ tsp. nutmeg
¼ tsp. ginger
3 T. cornstarch

¾ C. skim milk
1¼ C. canned or mashed
  cooked pumpkin
3 egg whites
⅓ C. granulated sugar
1-9" pie shell, baked

In saucepan, combine brown sugar, gelatin, salt and spices. Combine cornstarch and milk; stir until mixture comes to a boil. Remove from heat and stir in pumpkin. Chill until mixture mounds slightly when spooned. (Test every now and then - don't let it get too stiff.) Beat egg whites until soft peaks form; gradually add granulated sugar, beating to stiff peaks. Fold pumpkin mixture thoroughly into egg whites. Turn into crust. Chill firm.

QUICK STRAWBERRY BLENDER PIE

½ C. boiling water
1 pkg. strawberry jello
1 C. frozen strawberries,
  slightly thawed
½ C. crushed ice

2 T. lemon juice
2 T. non-fat dry milk
1-9" pie shell, baked
  or 6 tart shells, baked

Put boiling water and jello in blender and blend. Add remaining ingredients and blend (on and off a couple of times). Pour into baked pie shell. Garnish with special whipped topping and whole strawberries. (Very good and also very colorful!)

REFRESHING STRAWBERRY SHERBET

1-12 oz. pkg. frozen
strawberries
1-3 oz. pkg. strawberry gelatin
1/8 tsp. salt

1 C. boiling water
1 C. strawberry juice
 and water
1 C. evaporated skim milk

Thaw the frozen strawberries. Drain the strawberries and reserve their juice. Dissolve the strawberry gelatin and salt in the boiling water. Stir to dissolve the gelatin. Combine strawberry juice with enough water to yield 1 cup, add it to the gelatin and chill until slightly syrupy. Add milk gradually, stirring constantly and pour into shallow metal pan. Add strawberries and mix lightly. Place sherbet in freezer and freeze quickly until firm around the edges. Beat hard with a spoon. Return to the freezer and freeze until firm. Pack in a plastic container with a tight lid and leave in the freezer until ready to serve. If you are going to freeze this in a mechanical freezer, do not add the strawberries until the sherbet is starting to get firm. Yields: 1 quart of sherbet.

RICE KRISPIE COOKIES

1 C. margarine
½ C. egg substitute
1 C. brown sugar
1 C. white sugar
1 tsp. soda

½ tsp. cream of tartar
2 C. flour
2 C. oatmeal
2 C. Rice Krispies

Mix all ingredients, except oatmeal and Rice Krispies, well. Mix together oatmeal and Rice Krispies and fold into other ingredients. Drop by teaspoonful onto greased cookie sheet. Bake at 375° for 12 to 14 minutes. You can add raisins or nuts, if desired.

RICE KRISPIE MARSHMALLOW COOKIES

3 T. safflower oil
40 regular size marshmallows

½ tsp. vanilla
4 C. Rice Krispies

Warm the oil and add marshmallows, cooking over medium heat just until marshmallows are melted, stirring constantly. Add vanilla and pour in cereal. Mix well and drop by teaspoonfuls onto a sheet of waxed paper.

SHORTCAKES

2 C. sifted flour
¼ tsp. salt
1 T. baking powder
2 T. sugar

2 egg whites
⅓ C. oil
½ C. skim milk

Sift flour, salt, baking powder and sugar. Beat the egg whites and oil in a measuring cup. Add enough of the milk, or more if necessary to make 1 cup liquid. Add to the flour mixture. Mix with a fork until a dough is formed. Knead on a piece of waxed paper until smooth. Roll out to a thickness of ½". Cut with a 2" cookie cutter. Arrange on a baking sheet. Bake in a preheated 450° oven 12 minutes. Split with a fork while warm. Spread sliced strawberries or peaches between the layers. Top with mixture of fruit and vanilla yogurt.

SINGLE CRUST PASTRY SHELL

1 C. all-purpose flour
¼ tsp. salt
2 T. plus 2 tsp. vegetable
  shortening

2 T. plus 2 tsp. liquid
  Butter Buds
1 T. cold water

In mixing bowl, combine flour and salt. Cut in shortening, using a pastry blender or two knives, until mixture is the size of small peas. Add Butter Buds and mix lightly with fork. Add water, 1 teaspoon at a time, until dough is just moist enough to hold together. Form a ball. On floured surface, with floured rolling pin, roll dough out to a circle 1" larger than inverted 8 or 9" pie pan, fold pastry in half and transfer to pie pan; unfold and fit loosely into pan, gently patting out any air pockets. Makes 8 servings.

Unbaked Pastry Shell: Prepare single crust as directed. Fold edges to form a standing rim; flute. Pour in filling and bake as directed in recipe.

Baked Pastry Shell: Preheat oven to 450°. Prepare as directed for unbaked pastry shell. Prick bottom and sides with fork. Bake for 8 to 10 minutes or until lightly golden brown. Cool.

VANILLA ICE CREAM

2 C. skim milk
1 env. unflavored gelatin
1¼ C. sugar

2 C. skim evaporated milk
1½ tsp. vanilla

Heat skim milk to scalding point; do not boil. Remove from heat. Add gelatin and sugar. Mix until dissolved. Put into blender. Whirl 3 to 5 minutes. Add evaporated milk, whirl 2 minutes. Chill 5 hours or overnight. Process in ice cream freezer according to manufacturer's directions. Stir in vanilla. Chill 30 to 60 minutes.

YELLOW CUPCAKES

1 C. sifted flour	½ C. sugar
⅛ tsp. salt	1 tsp. vanilla extract
1 tsp. baking powder	¼ C. skim milk
¼ C. egg substitute	¼ C. oil

Blend flour, salt and baking powder. Beat the egg substitute, then gradually beat in the sugar until light and fluffy. Stir in the vanilla. Beat the milk and oil until creamy. Add to the egg mixture alternately with the flour mixture, beating until smooth after each addition. Spoon into lightly oiled and flour dusted pans. Bake in a preheated 350° oven for 20 minutes. Cool for 10 minutes.

ZUCCHINI COCOA CAKE

2½ C. whole wheat flour
2½ tsp. baking powder
1½ tsp. baking soda
½ C. cocoa
1 tsp. salt
1 tsp. cinnamon

¼ C. soft margarine
2 tsp. vanilla
2 C. ground zucchini
2 C. honey
¾ C. egg substitute
⅓ C. skim milk

Stir together dry ingredients. Put remaining ingredients in bowl, stir, then beat for 3 minutes. Combine bowl mixture with dry ingredients. Bake in a 9x12" greased pan at 350° for 35 to 40 minutes. Test with toothpick. Frost cake after it is cool.